Rx Shorthand

Rx Shorthand

Compiled and edited by

STANLEY JABLONSKI

ELSEVIER

Publisher: *HANLEY & BELFUS, INC.*
                  An Affiliate of Elsevier
                  1600 John F. Kennedy Boulevard
                  Philadelphia, PA 19103-2899

R$_x$ **Shorthand**   ISBN 1-56053-167-3

© 2005 Elsevier, Inc. All rights reserved.

© 1996 Hanley & Belfus, Inc.

No part of this book may be reproduced, reused, republished, or transmitted in any form or by any means without written permission of the publisher. Library of Congress Catalog card number 95-81921

Last digit is the print number: 9 8 7 6 5 4 3 2 1

Printed in Canada

A Historical Note

The recorded history of written prescriptions can be traced to ancient Egypt. One of the earliest known prescriptions is the Ebert Papyrus believed to have been written about 1500 B.C., which was discovered by Georg Ebers, German Egyptologist who lived from 1837 to 1898. Probably as old, if not older, is an ancient stone tablet, now in the collections of the New York Metropolitan Museum, on which there is carved the prescription for the preparation of fumigation, or vapor, for inhalation used by ancient physicians in the treatment of diseases.

The writings of ancient Greek physicians, particularly those of Hippocrates of Cos (physician who lived from c. 460 to c. 375 B.C.), who is considered by historians to be the "Father of Medicine," and Galen (Greek physician in Rome, whose name was Latinized to Claudius or Clarissimus Galenus, 131–203 A.D.) provide further examples of early prescriptions for medicinal preparations. Greek physicians usually followed the conservative hippocratic methods of treating disease; that is, mainly by appropriate diets and adjustment in patients' living style. Whenever these methods failed, however, medicinal preparations were prescribed that were compounded mostly from plant leaves, roots, and bark, the kinds and amounts of ingredients being specified. Medications compounded in accordance with the general principles of Galen's prescriptions are still in use in some parts of the world and are referred to as "galenicals."

As with most things in Western Civilization, the Renaissance was the turning point in the history of pharmacy. To a very large degree, the redirection of pharmacy after the Renaissance took place as a result of an innovative approach to compounding medicines introduced by Paracelsus, a Swiss physician born Aureolus Theophrastus Bombastus von Hohenheim, who lived from 1493 to 1541. Paracelsus was known to his contemporaries mainly for his unconventional lifestyle and manners; he was also a brilliant scientist who, by using his experience in alchemy, applied the principles of chemical synthesis to the production of medicinal preparations, thus laying the foundation on which the modern pharmaceutical industry is based.

Well into the 18th century, European physicians compounded medications themselves, but some hired apprentices to whom they relegated the preparation of medications, as well as minor surgical operations. Many former apprentices went on to open their own apothecaries from which they supplied physicians and surgeons (including their mentors) with crude ingredients, also dispensing some prescription medicines directly to patients. The apothecaries of the period thus served mainly as supply houses from which physicians purchased raw materials from which they themselves compounded prescription medicines.

The history of American pharmacy took a somewhat different course. There were not many physicians and pharmacists among the early settlers in the New World, and some of the physicians who did come to America combined the responsibilities of treating patients with compounding medicines used in their treatment out of necessity. Most early American pharmacies were thus owned and operated by physicians. The later waves of immigrants, however, did include some trained apothecaries. They usually opened their own shops, similarly to their European counterparts, mainly to serve as supply houses for physicians, but also dispensed prescription medicines as needed. Coincidentally, there was an increasingly popular view among contemporary American physicians that the responsibility for preparing and dispensing drugs should be turned over entirely to properly trained pharmacists. The leading advocate of this view was

John Morgan, a Philadelphia physician who lived from 1735 to 1789. The foundation of the Pharmaceutical Association and the Philadelphia College of Pharmacy in the mid-19th century marks the establishment of American pharmacy as an independent discipline within the realm of biomedical sciences with its own professional standards, educational requirements, and code of ethics.

From the middle of the 19th century on, American apothecaries underwent considerable changes, expanding their inventories to include prepared medications, patent medicines, nostrums, and later over-the-counter drugs.

General merchandise was eventually added to the shelves and, in time, many pharmacies installed lunch counters and soda fountains for the convenience of their customers, thus establishing the unique concept of the American drugstore.

The role of the pharmacist has also changed. Whereas before World War II, more than half of all prescriptions were compounded by the pharmacists, fewer than 1 in 100 prescriptions now require individual compounding. Pharmacists now turn their attention to patient education to ensure that prescribed medications are used properly, will not interfere with diagnostic tests, have no adverse effects on the fetus and newborn child, are compatible with other medications taken by the patient, and have no other potentially harmful influences.

The mortar and pestle, once the essential tools in the hands of pharmacists and the symbols of the profession, have little or no practical use in modern pharmacies.

The Prescription

Definition of Terms

addictive drug   see *drug, addictive*

adjuvant   (Lat. *adjuvans,* aiding) a substance that aids another substance, having no medicinal properties of its own, such as one that enhances the action of an active agent in a medicinal preparation

basis   the active substance in a medicinal preparation

brand name   see *name, proprietary*

compounded prescription   see *prescription, compounded*

controlled substance   see *substance, controlled*

corrective   (Lat. *corrigere,* to straighten, to correct) a substance that modifies undesirable properties of the basis or adjuvant in a medicinal preparation, as when eliminating an unpleasant taste

drug   1. any chemical substance used in the treatment, diagnosis, or prevention of disease
2. a narcotic agent or any substance that causes stupor
3. any addicting substance

drug, addictive   a drug, the repeated use of which may result in heavy dependence or addiction. Potentially addictive drugs used in the treatment of diseases are dispensed by prescription. Called also *habit-forming drug.*

drug, generic   see *name, generic*

drug, habit-forming   see *drug, addictive*

drug, hypnotic   a drug that may induce sleep. Hypnotic drugs are dispensed by prescription.

drug, legend   see *drug, prescription*

drug, nonlegend   see *drug, over-the-counter*

drug, nonprescription   see *drug, over-the-counter*

drug, nonproprietary   see *name, generic*

drug, over-the-counter (OTC)   a drug determined by the Food and Drug Administration (FDA) to be safe for use in self-medication and thus not required by law to be labeled with the R_x legend **"Caution: Federal Law Prohibits Dispensing Without Prescription,"** which may be dispensed without a prescription; hence the synonym *nonlegend drug*. Called also *nonprescription drug*.

drug, prescription   a drug that may be hypnotic, habit-forming, toxic, or otherwise potentially harmful and is not safe in self-medication; thus it is required by law to be dispensed only on prescription. Prescription drugs are sometimes referred to as *legend drugs* in that their containers are required by law to have imprinted the R_x legend, **"Caution: Federal Law Prohibits Dispensing Without Prescription."**

drug, proprietary   see *name, proprietary*

excipient   a substance that has no medicinal properties of its own and is added to a medication to stabilize its consistency or facilitate its administration, such as a solvent used to dilute a medication for intravenous administration or a base for an ointment. Called also *vehicle*.

generic drug, equivalency, name   see *name, generic*

habit-forming drug   see *drug, addictive*

hypnotic   see *drug, hypnotic*

inscription   (Lat. *in*, within + *scribere*, to write) the main part of a prescription containing the names and amounts of the prescribed ingredients

legend drug see *drug, prescription*

name, brand   see *name, proprietary*

name, generic   a nonproprietary name of a drug, usually descriptive of its chemical properties, that is not a protected trademark. Called also *generic drug, generic equivalency, nonproprietary drug, nonproprietary name, public name*.

name, proprietary   a name owned by a manufacturer of a drug and protected as to name, composition, and other properties by a trademark. Called also *brand name, proprietary drug, trademark name, trade name.*

name, public   see *name, generic*

name, trade   see *name, proprietary*

name, trademark   see *name, proprietary*

nonlegend drug   see *drug, over-the-counter*

nonprescription drug   see *drug, over-the-counter*

nonproprietary drug, name   see *name, generic*

OTC   see *drug, over-the-counter*

over-the-counter drug   see *drug, over-the-counter*

PPI   see *prepared patient package insert*

prepared patient package insert (PPI)   a package issued with certain prescription drugs containing information regarding the usefulness and potential side effects of the medication

prescription   (Lat. *praescriptio,* preamble) a written order for one or more medicinal agents, together with direction to the pharmacist for their preparation and the patient for their use. Sometimes used to mean *prescription drug* (see under *drug*).

prescription, compounded   a prescription requiring the pharmacist to mix the ingredients

prescription drug   see under *drug*

proprietary drug   see *name, proprietary*

public name   see *name, generic*

R$_x$ (Lat. *recipe,* take; the symbol is believed to have been originally *Rc*) a symbol representative of both the prescription and pharmacy. Also called *superscription.*

R$_x$ legend   see *drug, prescription*

S   see *signatura*

sig   see *signatura*

sign   see *signatura*

signatura   (Lat., the matrix of a seal) the part of a prescription containing the directions for the patient's use of the prescribed medication. Sometimes written in the English version.

signature   Abbreviated *S, sig,* or *sign.*

subscription   (Lat. *sub-,* under + *scribere,* to write) the part of a prescription containing dispensing directions to the pharmacist. In older prescriptions, the subscription served to give the directions for compounding of the prescribed medication; now the subscription is used mainly to designate the dosage form (tablets, capsules, ointment, and the like) and the number of dosage units to be supplied.

substance, controlled a drug, having a potential for abuse, controlled under special regulations of the Food and Drug Administration. Controlled substances used in the treatment of diseases are dispensed only by prescription.

superscription (Lat. *super-*, above + *scribere,* to write) see R_X.

trade name, trademark name see *name, proprietary*

vehicle See *excipient*

The Prescription Form

With the removal of the pharmacy from the doctor's office, physicians could no longer verbally instruct apothecaries on how to compound the medication they prescribed. This made it necessary that a standard form be devised for a physician to instruct a pharmacist about how the medication should be prepared. The first written prescription in America is believed to be that of Abraham Chovet, a Jamaican-born physician in Philadelphia. By the end of the 18th century, the use of the written prescription became universal in America.

A prescription is a written direction for the preparation and administration of medication or a special treatment, which may be issued by a physician, dentist, or other practitioner licensed by the state to prescribe drugs, including a podiatrist, osteopathic physician, physician's assistant, and nurse practitioner.

"Prescription" originates from Latin *praescriptio,* meaning preamble, rule, precept. In other European languages, terms meaning "prescription" are derived from a different Latin word, *recipere,* meaning to take, to receive, and include German *Rezept,* French *recette,* Italian *ricette,* and Polish *recepta. Recipe* (Latin imperative of *recipere*) is a source of the English symbol R_x (originally **Rc**), which identifies the rubric **superscription** on the prescription form; the Anglicized version, **recipe,** denotes directions for the preparation of something, mainly food, and has nothing to do with prescribing medicines.

Most prescription forms (or blanks) are imprinted with the name, address, the telephone number and other pertinent information, such as the name of a clinic or hospital. Other rubrics are as follows:

1. **Patient information**

   Includes the full name and address of the patient. Some prescription blanks, particularly those used by specialists such as pediatricians, include a space for the patient's age and/or weight to ensure proper dosage.

2. **Date**

   The dates of issue and filling the prescription are both listed. The law specifies that no prescription order for controlled substances may be dispensed or renewed more than 6 months after the date of issue of the prescription.

3. **R** (symbol for **superscription**)

   The symbol of both the prescription and pharmacy.

4. **Inscription** (medication prescribed)

   A rubric in which the names and quantities of the pre-scribed ingredients are identified. The manufacturer's proprietary (trademark) name may be indicated, requir-ing the pharmacist to dispense the product as indicated by the prescriber. Compounded prescriptions (those requir-ing the pharmacist to mix appropriate ingredients) list the names of individual names and amounts of ingredi-ents in either the metric or apothecary system of weights.

5. **Subscription** (dispensing direction to pharmacist)

   In older prescriptions, this rubric was reserved for direc-tions to the pharmacist for compounding the prescrip-tion. Now it is used mainly to designate the dosage form (tablets, caplets, capsules, etc.) and the number of dosage units to be dispensed.

6. **Signatura** (directions for patients to be placed on label)

   A rubric containing instructions for the proper use of the medication, usually written in Latin abbreviations which are translated for patients by the pharmacist into common English. Some prescription drugs are supplied with prepared patient package inserts (PPIs) containing information regarding the proper use of the drug, as well as its potential hazards.

7. **Refill**

The number of times the prescription may be refilled

8. **Prescriber signature**

As was customary in scientific and professional writings of the past, early prescriptions were written entirely in Latin. Even as late as 1921, Cary Eggleston devoted more than one-third of his book, *Essentials of Prescription Writing*, to the elements of the Latin grammar to ensure that prescriptions were written in the proper Latin form. Latin words and phrases used in prescriptions became abbreviated in time, evolving into a shorthand that became a private medium of communication between physicians and pharmacists, forming a language that is both precise and economical but is difficult for outsiders to decipher—even those with a good background in the classical languages—and is virtually incomprehensible to those who never studied Latin. As examples, **sos** is not a cry for help, as one could assume, but an abbreviation for Latin *si opus sit,* meaning "if it is necessary," and **sin** has nothing to do with transgression of religious laws, but is an abbreviation of Latin *sex in nocte,* meaning [take the medicine] "six times a night."

In the past, most prescriptions were **compounded**; that is, they contained directions for compounding the prescribed medication. Typically, a compounded prescription consists of four parts in the **inscription**:

1. **basis**   the active substance

2. **adjuvant**   a substance that has no medicinal properties of its own but is added to the medication to enhance the action of the basis

3. **corrective**   a substance that has no medicinal properties of its own but is added to the medication to correct and overcome undesired actions of the basis

Sample Prescription Form

JULIE F. LOCK-WESSON, M.D.
General Health Care
General Hospital
Philadelphia, PA 19000

215/000-1179

DEA# BZ 0000000
LIC.# MD 000000-E (PA)

NAME _Joe Jones_   AGE _43_

ADDRESS _Philadelphia PA_   DATE _9/29/05_

R

     Augmentin XR Tabs
     sig: Take 2 Tabs Q12 at the
     start of a meal for 10 days
     disp: 40 Tabs

REFILL _____ TIMES

☑ LABEL

Julie Lock-Wesson MD

Please see accompanying Prescribing Information

4. **excipient** a substance that has no medicinal properties of its own but is added to the medication to add bulk, stabilize its consistency, or facilitate its administration

The basis is always written in full but other ingredients may be identified by abbreviations:

aq dest (Latin *aqua destillata*) distilled water

spt (Latin *spiritus*) alcohol

suc (Latin *succus*) juice

nm (Latin *nux moschata*) nutmeg

Directions to the pharmacist (**subscription**) are generally written in shorthand expressions:

ft suppos (Latin *fiat suppositorium*) let suppository be made

m et sig (Latin *misce et signa*) mix and label

ad gr gust (*ad gradum gustum*) to agreeable taste

Directions for the patient (**signatura**) are prescribed by physicians in abbreviated Latin forms and are translated on labels by pharmacists into English:

alt dieb (Latin *alternis diebus*) translated on label as "every other day"

po (Latin *per os*) translated on label as "by mouth"

q2h (Latin *quaque secunda hora*) translated on label as "every two hours"

tid (Latin *ter in die*) translated on label as "three times a day"

Within the memory of older physicians and pharmacists who are still in practice, most prescription medicines were compounded in pharmacies. By using the R_X shorthand, physicians passed on to pharmacists coded instructions on how they wanted prescribed medications compounded, which active substances were to be used and in what amounts, what kind of excipients were permitted, which reagents were to be applied, how the medication should be taken by the patients, and some even adding an occasional admonition, such as reminding the pharmacist that the compounding should be done "according to the rules of art" (**sal** which is an abbreviation for Latin *secundum artis leges*)**,** or "let it be made skillfully" (**fsa** which is an abbreviation for Latin *fiat secundum artem*).

Prescriptions are no longer mixed manually; nearly all are filled with precompounded and prepackaged medications, and only very few require any individual compounding by the pharmacist, thus eliminating the need for compounding instruction, such as those which were routinely given under the rubric **subscription** in older prescriptions. The directions under the rubric **signatura,** in which patients are instructed how the prescribed medication should be taken, remain unchanged in prescription writing.

The glossary of Latin abbreviations lists those that are still in use, as well as those that were used in the past for directing pharmacists on compounding prescription drugs. Although the latter no longer have practical application in prescription writing they may be of importance to individuals who are interested in the history of pharmacy.

References

1. An Introduction to FDA Drug Regulation: A Manual for Pharmacists. Rockville, MD, Food and Drug Administration, 1990.
2. Approved Prescription Drug Products with Therapeutic Equivalence Evaluations. 8th ed. Washington, DC, US Dept. Health & Human Services, 1988.
3. Code of Federal Regulations, Title 21, 1300. Washington, DC, US Government Printing Office.
4. Eggleston G. Essentials of Prescription Writing. Philadelphia, W. B. Saunders, 1921.
5. Gennaro AR. Remington's Pharmaceutical Sciences. Easton, PA, Mack, 1990.
6. Jablonski S. Dictionary of Medical Acronyms and Abbreviations. 2nd ed. Philadelphia, Hanley & Belfus, 1993.
7. LaWall CH. Four Thousand Years of Pharmacy. Philadelphia, J. B. Lippincott, 1927.

8. Leake CD. An Historical Account of Pharmacology to the 20th Century. Springfield, Charles C. Thomas, 1975.
9. Smith CM, Reynard AM. Textbook of Pharmacology. Philadelphia, W. B. Saunders, 1992.
10. The R_X Legend: An FDA Manual for Pharmacists. Rockville, MD, US Food and Drug Administration, 1969.
11. The United States Pharmacopeia (USP 23). The National Formulary (NF) 18. Rockville, MD, United States Pharmacopeial Convention, 1995.

Acknowledgments

I wish to express my appreciation to members of the staff of the National Library of Medicine for their help in tracing and properly identifying a frequently elusive array of Latin abbreviations used in prescription writing. My special thanks go to Eve-Marie Lacroix, Lillian Scanlon, Robert Mehnert, and Dr. Maria Farkas.

I would also like to acknowledge the generous assistance received from Kathleen McCullough and Roberta Alberding.

My appreciation for making my book a reality goes to Hanley & Belfus Company and, especially, to Linda Belfus, whose comments and constructive suggestions were essential in putting together this book.

LATIN-ENGLISH DICTIONARY

A

A (Lat. *aqua*) water

aa (Lat. *ana*) so much of each

abs feb (Lat. *absente febre*) while fever is absent

an & hs (Lat. *ante cibum & hora somni*) before meals and at bedtime

ac (Lat. *ante cibum* sing.; *ante cibos* pl.) before meal(s)

ad (Lat. *adde*) add

add (Lat. *adde)* add

add c trit (Lat. *adde cum tritu*) add trituration

ad def an (Lat. *ad defectionen animi*) to the point of fainting

ad deliq (Lat. *ad deliquium*) to fainting

addend (Lat. *addendus*) to be added

ad effect (Lat. *ad effectum*) until effective

ad feb (Lat. *adstante febre*) fever being present

ad gr acid (Lat. *ad gratum aciditatem*) to an agreeable acidity

ad gr gust (Lat. *ad gratum gustum*) to an agreeable taste

adhib (Lat. *adhibentus*) to be administered

ad lib (Lat. *ad libitum*) as desired

admov, admove (Lat. *admoveatur*) apply, let there be applied

ad naus (Lat. *ad nauseam)* to the point of producing nausea

ad neut (Lat. *ad neutralizandum)* to neutralization

ad pond om (Lat. *ad pondus omnium)* to the weight of the whole

ad sat (Lat. *ad saturandum)* to saturation

adst feb (Lat. *adstante febre)* while fever is present

ad us (Lat. *ad usum)* according to custom

ad us ext (Lat. *ad usum externum*) for external use
ad 2 vic (Lat. *ad duas vices*) for two doses
adv (Lat. *adversum*) against
aet (Lat. *aetas*) age
ag feb (Lat. *aggrediente febre*) when the fever is coming on
agit (Lat. *agita*) shake
agit ant sum (Lat. *agita ante sumendum*) shake before taking
alb (Lat. *albus*) white
alt dieb (Lat. *alternis diebus*) every other day
alt hor (Lat. *alternis horis*) every other hour

B

b (Lat. *bis*) twice
BA (Lat. *balneum arenae*) sand bath
bal (Lat. *balneum*) bath
bd (Lat. *bis die*) twice a day
bds (Lat. *bis in die sumendus*) to be taken twice a day
ben (Lat. *bene*) well
bib (Lat. *bibe*) drink
bid (Lat. *bis in die*) twice a day
bihor (Lat. *bihorium*) during two hours
bin (Lat. *bis in nocte*) twice a night
bis (Lat. *bis*) twice
bm (Lat. *balneum maris*) salt water bath
bol (Lat. *bolus*) pill
bull (Lat. *bulliat*) let it boil
bv (Lat. *balneum vaporis*) steam bath

C

C (Lat. *centum*) one hundred
C (Lat. *congius*) gallon
c (Lat. *contusus*) bruised

c (Lat. *cibus*) meal

c (Lat. *compositus*) compound

c (Lat. *cum*) with

ca (Lat. *circa*) about

caf (Lat. *calefacio*) made warm

calef (Lat. *calefactus*) warmed

cap (Lat. *capiat*) take, let him (her) take

cap (Lat. *capsula*) capsule

capiend (Lat. *capiendus*) to be taken

cap moli (Lat. *capsula mollis*) soft capsule

cap quant vult (Lat. *capiat quantum vult*) to be taken as much as one wants to

cf (Lat. *confer*) compare

chart (Lat. *charta*) paper

chart cerat (Lat. *charta cerata*) waxed paper

cib (Lat. *cibus*) food

cit disp (Lat. *cito dispensetur*) dispense quickly, let it be dispensed quickly

cm (Lat. *cras mane*) tomorrow morning

cms (Lat. *cras mane sumendus*) to be taken tomorrow morning

cn (Lat. *cras nocte*) tomorrow night

cns (Lat. *cras nocte sumendus*) to be taken tomorrow night

co (Lat. *compositus*) compounded

cochl (Lat. *cochleare*) a spoonful

cochl amp (Lat. *cochleare amplum*) a healing spoonful

cochl inf (Lat. *cochleare infans*) a teaspoonful

cochl mag (Lat. *cochleare magnum*) a tablespoonful

cochl med (Lat. *cochleare medium*) a dessertspoonful

cochl parv (Lat. *cochleare parvum*) a teaspoonful

coct (Lat. *coctio*) boiling

colat (Lat. *colatus*) strained

colet (Lat. *coletur*) strain, let it be strained

coll (Lat. *collyrium*) eyewash

collut (Lat. *collutorium*) mouthwash

collyr (Lat. *collyrium*) eyewash

color (Lat. *coleretur*) color, let it be colored

con (Lat. *contra*) against

con (Lat. *congius*) gallon

concis (Lat. *concisus*) cut

cons (Lat. *conserva*) keep

consperg (Lat. *consperge*) sprinkle

cont (Lat. *contra*) against

cont (Lat. *contagio*) infection

cont (Lat. *contusus*) bruised

contag (Lat. *contagio*) infection

conter (Lat. *contere*) rub together

contin (Lat. *continuetur*) continue, let it be continued

cont rem (Lat. *continuetur remedium*) continue the medicine, let the medicine be continued

contrit (Lat. *contritus*) broken down

contus (Lat. *contusus*) bruised

coq (Lat. *coque*) boil

coq in s a (Lat. *coque in sufficiente aqua*) boil in sufficient water

coq s a (Lat. *coque secundum artem*) boil properly

cor (Lat. *corpus*) body

crast (Lat. *crastinus*) for tomorrow

cta (Lat. *catamenia*) menses

ctant (Lat. *cum tanto*) with the same amount

cuj (Lat. *cujus*) of which

cuj lib (Lat. *cujus liber*) of whatever you please

cum aq (Lat. *cum aqua*) with water

cyath (Lat. *cyathus*) a glassful

D

D (Lat. *dosis*) dose

d (Lat. *da*) give

d (Lat. *datur*) give, let it be given

d (Lat. *dexter*) right

d (Lat. *dies*) day

d (Lat. *dividetur*) divide, let it be divided

dand (Lat. *dandus*) to be given

dd (Lat. *de die*) daily

dd (Lat. *datur ad*) let it be given to

dd in d (Lat. *de die in diem*) from day to day

deb spis (Lat. *debita spissutudine*) of the proper consistency

decoct (Lat. *decoctum*) decoction

dec (Lat. *decanta*) pour off

decub (Lat. *decubitus*) laying down

de d in d (Lat. *de die in diem*) from day to day

deglut (Lat. *deglutiatur*) swallow, let it be swallowed

dent (Lat. *dentur*) give, let it be given

dent tal dos (Lat. *dentur tales doses*) give of such doses, let it be given of such doses

dep (Lat. *depuratus*) purified

dest (Lat. *destilla, destillatus*) distill, distilled

det (Lat. *detur*) give, let it be given

det in dup, det in 2 plo (Lat. *detur in duplo*) let twice as much be given

d et s (Lat. *detur et signetur*) give and label, let it be given and labeled

dex (Lat. *dexter*) right

dieb alt (Lat. *diebus alternis*) on alternate days

dieb tert (Lat. *diebus tertiis*) every third day

dig (Lat. *digeretur*) let it be digested

diluc (Lat. *diluculo*) at daybreak

dilut (Lat. *dilutus*) dilute, diluted

dim (Lat. *dimidus*) one half

d in p aeq (Lat. *dividetur in partes aequales*) divide into equal parts, let it be divided in equal parts

dir prop (Lat. *directione propria*) with proper direction

disp (Lat. *dispensa, dispensetur*) dispense, let it be dispensed

div (Lat. *divide, dividatur*) divide, let it be divided

dol (Lat. *dolor*) pain

dos (Lat. *dosis*) dose

dtd (Lat. *datur talis dosis, datur tales doses*) give such a dose, give such doses, let it be given in such doses

dup (Lat. *duplicitas*) doubling, duplication

dur (Lat. *duris*) hard

dur dol (Lat. *durante dolor*) while pain lasts

E

ead (Lat. *eadem*) the same

ejusd (Lat. *ejusdem*) of the same

elix (Lat. *elixir*) elixir

emp (Lat. *emplastrum*) plaster

emp (Lat. *ex modo prescripto*) as directed

emp vesic (Lat. *emplastrum vesicatorium*) blistering plaster

emul (Lat. *emulsum*) emulsion

es (Lat. *enema saponis*) soap enema

exhib (Lat. *exhibeatur*) give, let it be given

F

feb (Lat. *febris*) fever

feb dur (Lat. *febre durante*) while the fever lasts

ferv (Lat. *fervens*) boiling

fh (Lat. *fiat haustus*) let a draught be made

fla (Lat. *fiat lege artis*) let it be done according to the rule

flav (Lat. *flavus*) yellow

fm (Lat. *fiat mistura*) make a mixture

fol (Lat. *folium*) leaf

fort (Lat. *fortis*) strong

fp (Lat. *fiat potio*) let a potion be made

f pil (Lat. *fiat pilulae*) make pills, let pills be made

fract dos (Lat. *fracta dosi*) in divided doses

frig (Lat. *frigidus*) cold

frust (Lat. *frustillatim*) in small pieces

fsa (Lat. *fiat secundum artem*) make it skillfully, let it be made skillfully

fsar (Lat. *fiat secundum artem regulas*) make it according to the rules, let it be made according to the rules

ft (Lat. *fiat, fiant*) make, let there be made

ft cataplasm (Lat. *fiat cataplasma*) make a poultice, let a poultice be made

ft cerat (Lat. *fiat ceratum*) make a cerate, let a cerate be made

ft collyr (Lat. *fiat collyrium*) make an eyewash, let an eyewash be made

ft emuls (Lat. *fiat emulsio*) make an emulsion, let an emulsion be made

ft enem (Lat. *fiat enema*) make an enema, let an enema be made

ft garg (Lat. *fiat gargarisma*) make a gargle, let a gargle be made

ft infus (Lat. *fiat infusum*) make an injection, let an injection be made

ft linim (Lat. *fiat linimentum*) make a liniment, let a liniment be made

ft mas (Lat. *fiat massa*) make a mass, let a mass be made

ft mas div in pil (Lat. *fiat massa dividenda in pilulae*) make a mass and divide it into pills, let a mass be made and divide it into pills

ft mist (Lat. *fiat mistura*) make a mixture, let a mixture be made

ft pulv (Lat. *fiat pulvis*) make a powder, let a powder be made

ft solut (Lat. *fiat solutio*) make a solution, let a solution be made

ft suppos (Lat. *fiat suppositorium*) make a suppository, let a suppository be made

G

garg (Lat. *gargarisma*) gargle
gel (Lat. *gelatina*) jelly
gel quav (Lat. *gelatina quavis*) any kind of jelly
grad (Lat. *gradatim*) by degrees
grav (Lat. *gravitas*) pregnancy

gt (Lat. *gutta*) drop
gtt (Lat. *guttae*) drops
gutt (Lat. *gutturi*) to the throat
guttat (Lat. *guttatim*) drop by drop
gutt quibusd (Lat. *guttis quibusdam*) with a few drops

H

h (Lat. *haustus*) a draft
h (Lat. *hora*) hour
haust (Lat. *haustus*) a draft
hd (Lat. *hora decubitus*) at bedtime
hebdom (Lat. *hebdomas*) a week
hn (Lat. *hoc nocte*) tonight
hoc vesp (Lat. *hoc vespere*) this evening
hor (Lat. *hora*) hour
hora decub (Lat. *hora decubitus*) at bedtime
hor som (Lat. *hora somni*) at bedtime
hor un spatio (Lat. *horae unius spatio*) at the end of one hour
hor interm (Lat. *horis intermediis*) at intermediate hours
hs (Lat. *hora somni*) at bedtime
ht (Lat. *haustus*) a draught

I

ic (Lat. *inter cibos*) between meals
id (Lat. *idem*) the same
i d (Lat. *in diem*) during the day
idon vehic (Lat. *idoneo vehiculo*) in a suitable vehicle
illic (Lat. *illico*) immediately
in aq (Lat. *in aqua*) in water
in d (Lat. *in dies*) daily
inf (Lat. *infunde*) pour in
inj enem (Lat. *injiciatur enema*) inject an enema, let an enema be injected

in loc ferv (Lat. *in loco fervente*) in a hot place
in loc frig (Lat. *in loco frigido*) in a cold place
int cib (Lat. *inter cibos*) between meals
int noct (Lat. *inter noctem*) during the night
in vas claus (Lat. *in vaso clauso*) in a closed vessel
in vit (Lat. *in vitro*) in a glass

J

jentac (Lat. *jentaculum*) breakfast
juxt (Lat. *juxta*) near

L

l (Lat. *limen*) threshold
l (Lat. *limes*) boundary
la (Lat. *lege artis*) according to the art
laev (Lat. *laevus*) left
lag (Lat. *lagena*) flask
lapid (Lat. *lapideus*) of stone
lat dol (Lat. *lateri dolenti*) to the painful side
lev (Lat. *levis*) light
lin (Lat. *linimentum*) liniment
liq (Lat. *liquor*) liquid
loc dol (Lat. *loco dolenti*) to the painful side
lut (Lat. *luteus*) yellow
lot (Lat. *lotio*) lotion

M

m (Lat. *macerare*) macerate
m (Lat. *misce*) mix
mac (Lat. *macerare*) macerate

m accur (Lat. *misce accuratissime*) mix very accurately
mag (Lat. *magnus*) large
magn (Lat. *magnus*) large
man (Lat. *manipulus*) handful
man (Lat. *mane*) morning
manip (Lat. *manipulus*) handful
man pr (Lat. *mane primo*) early in the morning
mas pi (Lat. *massa pilularum*) pill mass
matut (Lat. *matutinus*) in the morning
mb (Lat. *misce bene*) mix well
m caute (Lat. *misce caute*) mix with caution
m dict (Lat. *modo dicto*) as directed
m et n (Lat. *mane et nocte*) morning and night
m et sig (Lat. *misce et signa*) mix and write a label
m ft (Lat. *mistura fiat*) let a mixture be made
mist (Lat. *mistura*) mixture
mit (Lat. *mitte*) sand
mod praes (Lat. *modo praescripto*) in the way directed
moll (Lat. *mollis*) soft
mor dict (Lat. *more dicto*) in the manner directed
mor sol (Lat. *more solito*) in the usual way
mp (Lat. *modo praescripto*) as directed
mtd (Lat. *mitte tales doses*) send such doses

N

nb (Lat. *nota bene*) note well
nebul (Lat. *nebula*) spray
n et m (Lat. *nocte et mane*) night and day
nl (Lat. *non liquet*) it is not clear
nl (Last. *non licet*) it is not permitted
nm (Lat. *nux moschata*) nutmeg
No (Lat. *numero*) number
no (Lat. *numero*) number
noc (Lat. *nocte*) night, at night
noct (Lat. *nocte*) night, at night
noct maneq (Lat. *nocte maneque*) at night and in the morning

non rep (Lat. *non repetatur*) do not repeat, let it not be repeated

non repetat (Lat. *non repetatur*) do not repeat, let it not be repeated

npo (Lat. *nulla per os*) nothing by mouth

npo/hs (Lat. *nulla per os hora somni*) nothing by mouth at bedtime

nr (Lat. *non repetatur*) do not repeat, let it not be repeated

O

o (Lat. *oculus*) eye

o (Lat. *octarius*) pint

od (Lat. *omni die*) daily

odorat (Lat. *odoratus*) odoriferous

oh (Lat. *omni hora*) every hour

ol (Lat. *oleum*) oil

om (Lat. *omni mane*) every morning

omn (Lat. *omni bihora*) every two hours

omn hor (Lat. *omni hora*) every hour

omn 2 hor (Lat. *omni secunda hora*) every second hour

omn man (Lat. *omni mane*) every morning

omn noct (Lat. *omni nocte*) every night

omn quad hor (Lat. *omni quadranta hora*) every quarter of an hour

omn quar hor (Lat. *omni quadranta hora*) every quarter of an hour

omn tert hor (Lat. *omni tertia hora*) every third hour

on (Lat. *omni nocte*) every night

ou (Lat. *oculus uterque*) each eye

P

p (Lat. *pondere*) by weight

p (Lat. *pugilus*) a handful

p ae (Lat. *partes aequales*) equal parts

par aff (Lat. *pars affecta*) the part affected

part aeq (Lat. *partes aequales*) equal parts

part dolent (Lat. *partes dolentes*) painful parts

part vic (Lat. *partitis vicibus*) in divided doses

pc (Lat. *post cibum, post cibos*) after meal(s)

per op emet (Lat. *peracta operatione emetici*) when the action of emetic is over

pil (Lat. *pilula*) pill

PM (Lat. *post meridiem*) after noon

po (Lat. *per os*) by mouth, orally, by way of the mouth

pocill (Lat. *pocillum*) small cup

pocul (Lat. *poculum*) cup

pond (Lat. *pondere*) by weight

post sing sed liq (Lat. *post singulus sedes liquidas*) after very loose stool

ppa (Lat. *phiala prius agitata*) first shake well

pr (Lat. *per rectum*) by rectum, rectally, by way of the rectum

p rat aetat (Lat. *pro ratione aetatis*) in proportion to age

prim luc (Lat. *prima luce*) first thing in the morning, at first light

prim m (Lat. *primo mane*) first thing in the morning

prn (Lat. *pro re nata*) as required

pro us ext (Lat. *pro uso externo*) for external use

pt (Lat. *perstetur*) let it be continued

pu (Lat. *per urethra*) by urethra, by way of the urethra

pulv (Lat. *pulvis*) powder

pulv gros (Lat. *pulvis grossus*) coarse powder

pulv subtil (Lat. *pulvis subtilis*) smooth powder

pulv tenu (Lat. *pulvis tenuis*) very fine powder

pv (Lat. *per vaginam*) by vagina, vaginally, by way of the vagina

Q

q (Lat. *quantum*) amount

q (Lat. *quaque*) each, every

qd (Lat. *quaque die*) every day

qds (Lat. *quater die sumendum*) to be taken four times a day

qh (Lat. *quaque hora*) every hour

q2h (Lat. *quaque secunda hora*) every second hour

q3h (Lat. *quaque tertia hora*) every third hour

q4h (Lat. *quaque quarta hora*) every fourth hour

qhs (Lat. *quaque hora somni*) every hour of sleep

qid (Lat. *quater in die*) four times a day

ql (Lat. *quantum libet)* as much as desired

qm (Lat. *quaque mane*) every morning

qn (Lat. *quaque nocte*) every night

quotid (Lat. *quotide*) daily

qp (Lat. *quantam placeat*) as much as desired

qPM (Lat. *quaque post meridiem*) every afternoon

qq (Lat. *quaque*) every

qqd (Lat. *quaque die*) every day

qqh (Lat. *quaque quarta hora*) every fourth hour

qq hor (Lat. *quaque hora*) every hour

qr (Lat. *quantum rectum*) correct quantity

qs (Lat. *quantum sufficit*) as much as will suffice

qs (Lat. *quantum satis*) sufficient quantity

q sat (Lat. *quantum satis*) sufficient quantity

q suff (Lat. *quantum sufficit*) as much as suffices

quat (Lat. *quattuor*) four

quinq (Lat. *quinque*) five

quotid (Lat. *quotidie*) daily

qv (Lat. *quantum vis*) as much as desired

R

redig in pulv (Lat. *redigatur in pulverem*) let it be reduced to powder

red in pulv (Lat. *reductus in pulverem*) reduced to powder

ren (Lat. *renovetur*) renew, let it be renewed

ren sem (Lat. *renovetum semel*) renew only once, let it be renewed only once

rep (Lat. *repetatur*) rcpcat, let it be repeated

rs (Lat. *rasurae*) scrapings or filings

rub (Lat. *ruber*) red

R (Lat. *recipe*) prescribe, prescription, prescription drug, take

S

s (Lat. *semis*) half

s (Lat. *sinister*) left

sa (Lat. *secundum artem*) according to art

sai (Lat. *sine altera indicatione*) without other qualifications

sal (Lat. *secundum artis leges*) according to the rules of art

sem (Lat. *semis*) one half

semih (Lat. *semihora*) half an hour

sept (Lat. *septem*) seven

ser (Lat. *serva*) serve, preserve

sesquih (Lat. *sesquihora*) an hour and a half

s expr (Lat. *sine expressio*) without expressing

sic (Lat. *siccus*) dry

sig (Lat. *signa, signetur*) let it be labeled

sig n pro (Lat. *signa nomine proprio*) label with the proper name

sin (Lat. *sine*) without

sin (Lat. *sex in nocte*) six times a night

sinap (Lat. *sinapis*) mustard

sin aq (Lat. *sine aqua*) without water

si non val (Lat. *si non valeat*) if it is not enough

si op sit (Lat. *si opus sit*) if it is necessary

si vir perm (Lat. *si vires permittant*) if the strength will permit

sl (Lat. *secundum legem*) according to the rules

sol (Lat. *solutio*) solution

solv (Lat. *solve*) dissolve

s op s (Lat. *si opus sit*) if it is necessary

sos (Lat. *si opus sit*) if it is necessary

sp (Lat. *spiritus*) alcohol

spir (Lat. *spiritus*) alcohol

spiss (Lat. *spissatus*) inspissated, thickened by evaporation

spt (Lat. *spiritus*) alcohol

ss (Lat. *semis*) one half

ssv (Lat. *sub signo veneni*) under a poison label

st (Lat. *stet*) let it stand

st (Lat. *stent*) let them stand

stat (Lat. *statim*) immediately

stillat (Lat. *stillatim*) drop by drop

su (Lat. *sumat*) let him take it

sub fin coct (Lat. *sub finem coctionis*) toward the end of boiling

suc (Lat. *succus*) juice

sum (Lat. *sumat*) let him take

sum (Lat. *sumendum*) to be taken

suppos (Lat. *suppositorium*) suppository

sv (Lat. *spiritus vini*) spirit of wine

svr (Lat. *spiritus vini rectificans*) rectified spirit of wine

syr (Lat. *syrupus*) syrup

T

tab (Lat. *tabella*) tablet

tal (Lat. *talis*) such a one

td (Lat. *ter die*) three times daily

tds (Lat. *ter die sumendum*) to be taken three times a day

tid (Lat. *ter in die*) three times a day

tin (Lat. *ter in nocte*) three times a night

tinc (Lat. *tinctura*) tincture

trid (Lat. *triduum*) three days

trit (Lat. *tritura*) triturate

troch (Lat. *trochiscus*) lozenge

tus (Lat. *tussis*) cough

U-Z

u (Lat. *utendus*) to be used
ud (Lat. *ut dictum*) as directed
ult praes (Lat. *ultimum praescriptus*) last prescribed
ung (Lat. *unguentum*) ointment
ut dict (Lat. *ut dictum*) as directed
utend (Lat. *utendus*) to be used
vesp (*vespera*) evening
vic (Lat. *vices*) times

ENGLISH-LATIN REVERSE DICTIONARY

A

about ca (Lat. *circa*)
according to art la (Lat. *lege artis*); sa (Lat. *secundum artem*)
according to custom ad us (Lat. *ad usum*)
according to rules sl (Lat. *secundum legem*)
according to rules of art sal (Lat. *ecundum artis leges*)
acidity see *to agreeable acidity*
add ad, add (Lat. *adde*)
  see also *to be added*
add trituration add c trit (Lat. *adde cum tritu*)
add water aq ad (Lat. *aquam ad*)
administer see *to be administered*
after meal(s) pc (Lat. *post cibum* sing.; *post cibos* pl.)
after noon PM (Lat. *post meridiem*)
  see also *every afternoon*
after very loose stools post sing set liq (Lat. *post singulus sedes liquidas*)
against adv (Lat. *adversum*); con (Lat. *contra*)
age aet (Lat. *aetas*)
  see also *in proportion to age*
alcohol sp, spt (Lat. *spiritus*)
amount q (Lat. *quantum*)
  see also *with the same amount*
antepartal AP, ap (Lat. *ante partum*)
any kind of jelly gel quav (Lat. *gelatina quavis*)
apply see *let there by applied*
ascribed to ascr (Lat. *ascriptum*)
as desired ad lib (Lat. *ad libitum*)
as directed ud (Lat. *ut dictum*); emp (Lat. *ex modo praescripto*); m dict (Lat. *modo dicto*); mod praes (Lat. *modo*

praescripto); mp (Lat. *modo praescripto*); ut dict (Lat. *ut dictum*)

as much as desired ql (Lat. *quantam libet*); qp (Lat. *quantam placeat*)

as much as you desire qv (Lat. *quantum vis*)

as much as will suffice qs (Lat. *quantum sufficit*)

as much as suffices q suff (Lat. *quantum sufficit*)

as required prn (Lat. *pro re nata*)

at bedtime hd (Lat. *hora decubitus*); hor decub (Lat. *hora decubitus*); hor som (Lat. *hori somni*); hs (Lat. *hora somni*)

at daybreak diluc (Lat. *diluculo*)

at end of one hour hor un spatio (Lat. *horae unius spatio*)

at first light see *first thing in the morning*

at intermediate hours hor interm (Lat. *horis intermediis*)

at night noc, noct (Lat. *nocte*)

at night and in the morning noct maneq (Lat. *nocte maneque*)

B

bath bal (Lat. *balneum*)
  see also *salt water bath*
  see also *sand bath*
  see also *steam bath*

bedtime hd, hor decub (Lat. *hora decubitus*); hs, hor som (Lat. *hora somni*)
  see also *at bedtime*
  see also *before meals and at bedtime*
  see also *nothing by mouth at bedtime*

before breakfast ant jetac (Lat. *ante jentaculum*)

before dinner ap (Lat. *ante prandium*)

before meal(s) ac (Lat. *ante cibum* sing.; *ante cibos* pl.)

before meals and at bedtime ac & hs (Lat. *ante cibum & hora somni*)

before noon AM, am (Lat. *ante meridiem*)

before parturition see *antepartal*

between meals ic, int cib (Lat. *inter cibos*)

blistering plaster emp vesic (Lat. *emplastrum vesicatorium*)
body cor (Lat. *corpus*)
boil coq (Lat. *coque*)
   see also *let it boil*
boil in sufficient water coq in s a (Lat. *coque in sufficiente aqua*)
boil properly coq s a (Lat. *coque secundum artem*)
boiling coct (Lat. *coctio*); ferv (Lat. *fervens*)
   see also *toward the end of boiling*
boiling water aq bull (Lat. *aqua bulliens*)
boundary l (Lat. *limes*)
breakfast jentac (Lat. *jentaculum*)
   see also *before breakfast*
broken down contrit (Lat. *contritus*)
bruised c, cont, contus (Lat. *contusus*)
by degrees grad (Lat. *gradatim*)
by mouth po (Lat. *per os*)
by rectum pr (Lat. *per rectum*)
by urethra pu (Lat. *per urethra*)
by vagina pv (Lat. *per vaginam*)
by way of mouth see *by mouth*
by way of rectum see *by rectum*
by way of urethra see *by urethra*
by way of vagina see *by vagina*
by weight p, pond (Lat. *pondere*)

C

capsule cap (Lat. *capsula*)
   see also *soft capsule*
cerate cerat (Lat. *ceratum*)
   see also *let cerate be made*
coarse powder pulv gros (Lat. *pulvis grossus*)
cold frig (Lat. *frigidus*)
cold water aq frig (Lat. *aqua frigata*)
color see *let it be colored*
compare cf (Lat. *confer*)

compound, compounded c, co (Lat. *compositus*)
constipation see *when the bowels are constipated*
continue see *let it be continued*
  see *let the medicine be continued*
cough tus (Lat. *tussis*)
cup pocul (Lat. *poculum*)
  see also *small cup*
custom see *according to custom*
cut concis (Lat. *concisus*)

D

daily dd (Lat. *de die*); die (Lat. *die*); in d (Lat. *in dies*); od
  (Lat. *omni die*); qd (Lat. *quaque die*); quotid (Lat. *quoti-*
  die)
day d (Lat. *dies*)
  see also *daily*
  see also *during the day*
  see also *every day*
  see also *every other day*
  see also *every third day*
  see also *four times daily*
  see also *from day to day*
  see also *night and day*
  see also *on alternate days*
  see also *three days*
  see also *three times a day*
  see also *three times daily*
  see also *to be taken four times a day*
  see also *to be taken three times a day*
  see also *twice a day*
daybreak see *at daybreak*
decoction decoct (Lat. *decoctum*)
degree see *by degrees*
dessertspoonful cochl med (Lat. *cochleare medium*)
digest see *let it be digested*

diluted dilut (Lat. *dilutus*)

dinner p (Lat. *prandium*)
  see also *before dinner*

directions see *as directed*
  see *in the manner directed*
  see *in the usual manner*
  see *in the way directed*
  see *with proper direction*

dispense disp (Lat. *dispensa, dispensetur*)

dispense quickly See *let it be dispensed quickly*

dissolve solv (Lat. *solve*)

distill, distilled dest (Lat. *destilla, destillatus*)

discharge from the bowels alv deject (Lat. *alvi dejectiones*)

dispense see *let it be dispensed*

distilled water aq dest (Lat. *aqua destillata*)

divide see *let it be divided*

divide into equal parts see *let it be divided into equal parts*

do not repeat see *let it not be repeated*

dose D, dos (Lat. *dosis*)
  see also *for two doses*
  see also *give of such dose(s)*
  see also *in divided doses*
  see also *send such doses*

doubling, duplication dup (Lat. *duplicitas*)

draft h, haust, ht (Lat. *haustus*)
  see also *let a draught be made*

drink bib (Lat. *bibe*)

drop gt (Lat. *gutta*)

drop by drop guttat (Lat. *guttatim*); stillat
  (Lat. *stillatim*)

drops gtt (Lat. *guttae*)
  see also *with a few drops*

dry sic (Lat. *siccus*)

during the night int noct (Lat. *inter noctem*)

during two hours bih (Lat. *bihorium*)

E

each q (Lat. *quaque*); o, omn (Lat. *omni*)
  see also *every*
  see also *so much of each*
each ear au (Lat. *auris uterque*)
each eye ou (Lat *oculus uterque*)
early in the morning man pr (Lat. *mane primo*)
effective see *until effective*
elixir elix (Lat. *elixir*)
emetic see *when the action of emetic is over*
emulsion emul (Lat. *emulsum*)
  see also *let emulsion be made*
enema enem (Lat. *enema*)
  see also *let enema be injected*
  see also *let enema be made*
  see also *soap enema*
equal a, ae (Lat. *aequalis* sing.; *aequales* pl.)
equal parts ae, part aeq (Lat. *partes aequales*)
evening vesp (Lat. *vespere*)
  see also *this evening*
every q, qq (Lat. *quaque*); o, omn (Lat. *omni*)
  see also *each*
every afternoon qPM (Lat. *quaque post meridiem*)
every day qd, qqd (Lat. *quaque die*)
every fourth hour qqh, q4r (Lat. *quaque quarta hora*)
every hour oh, omn hor (Lat. *omni hora*); qh, qqr (Lat. *quaque hora*)
every hour of sleep qhs (Lat. *quaque hora somni*)
every morning omn man, om (Lat. *omni mane*); qm (Lat. *quaque mane*)
every night omn, on (Lat. *omni nocte*); qn (Lat. *quaque nocte*)
every other day alt dieb (Lat. *alternis diebus*)
every other hour alt hor (Lat. *alternis horis*)
every other night alt noct (Lat. *alternis nocte*)

every quarter of an hour omn quad hor, omn quar hor
(Lat. *omni quadranta hora*)

every second hour omn 2 hor (Lat. *omni secunda hora*)

every third day dieb tert (Lat. *diebus tertiis*)

every third hour omn tert hor, q3h (Lat. *omni tertia hora,
quaque tertia hora*)

every two hours omn bih (Lat. *omni bihora*); q2h (Lat.
quaque secunda hora)

external use see *for external use*

eye o (Lat. *oculus*)
see also *each eye*

eyewash coll, collyr (Lat. *collyrium*)
see also *let eyewash be made*

F

fainting see *to fainting*
see *to the point of fainting*

fever feb (Lat. *febris*)

fever being present ad feb (Lat. *adstante febre*)
see also *when fever is coming on*
see also *while fever is absent*
see also *while fever is present*
see also *while fever lasts*

first shake well ppa (Lat. *phiala prius agitata*)

first thing in the morning prim luc (Lat. *prima luce*); prim
m (Lat. *primo mane*)

five quinq (Lat. *quinque*)

flask lag (Lat. *lagena*)

food cib (Lat. *cibus*)

for external use ad us ext (Lat. *ad usum externum*); pro us
ext (Lat. *pro uso externo*)

for tomorrow crast (Lat. *crastinus*)

for two doses ad 2 vic (Lat. *duas vices*)

four quat (Lat. *quattuor*)

four times daily qid (Lat. *quater in die*)

from day to day dd in d, de d in d (Lat. *de die in diem*)

G

gallon C, con (Lat. *congius*)
gargle garg (Lat. *gargarisma*)
  see also *let gargle be made*
ginger zz (Lat. *zingibar*)
give see *let it be given*
  see *to be given*
give of such dose(s) see *let it be given of such dose(s)*
  see *let it be given*
  see *let be given to*
  see *to be given*
glassful cyath (Lat. *cyathus*)

H

half dim (Lat. *dimidus*); s, sem, ss (Lat. *semis*)
half an hour semih (Lat. *semihora*)
handful man, manip (Lat. *manipulus*); p (Lat. *pugilus*)
hard dur (Lat. *duris*)
heaping spoonful cochl amp (Lat. *cochleare amplum*)
hot water aq cal (Lat. *aqua calida*); aq ferv (Lat. *aqua fervens*)
hour h, hor (Lat. *hora*)
  see also *at end of one hour*
  see also *at intermediate hours*
  see also *during two hours*
  see also *every fourth hour*
  see also *every hour*
  see also *every hour of sleep*
  see also *every other hour*
  see also *every quarter of an hour*
  see also *every second hour*
  see also *every third hour*
  see also *every two hours*
  see also *half an hour*

I

if it is necessary s op s, si op sit, sos (Lat. *si opus sit*)
if it is not enough si no val (Lat. *si non valeat*)
if the strength will permit si vir perm (Lat. *si vires permitant*)
immediately illic (Lat. *illico*); stat (Lat. *statim*)
in a closed vessel in vas claus (Lat. *in vaso clauso*)
in a cold place in loc frig (Lat. *in loco frigido*)
in divided doses fract dos (Lat. *fracta dosi*); part vic (Lat. *partitiss vicibus*)
in a glass in vit (Lat. *in vitro*)
in a hot place in loc ferv (Lat. *in loco fervente*)
in the manner directed mor dict (Lat. *more dicto*)
in the morning matut (Lat. *matutinus*)
in proportion to age p rat aetat (Lat. *pro ratione aetatis*)
in small pieces frust (Lat. *frustillatim*)
in a suitable vehicle idon vehic (Lat. *idoneo vehiculo*)
in the usual manner moe aol (Lat. *more solito*)
in the way directed see *as directed*
in water in aq (Lat. *in aqua*)
in the way directed mod praes (Lat. *modo praescipto*)
increase aug (Lat. *augere*)
infection cont, contag (Lat. *contagio*)
injection see *let injection be made*
inspissated spiss (Lat. *spissatus*)
it is not clear nl (Lat. *non liquet*)

J–K

jelly gel (Lat. *gelatina*)
  see also *any kind of jelly*
juice suc (Lat. *succus*)
keep cons (Lat. *conserva*); ser (Lat. *serva*)

L

label see *let it be given and labeled*
   see *let it be labeled*
   see *mix and write label*
   see *under poison label*
label with proper name sig n pro (Lat. *signa nomine proprio*)
large mag, magn (Lat. *magnus*)
last prescribed ult praes (Lat. *ultimum praescriptus*)
leaf fol (Lat. *folium*)
left laev (Lat. *laevus*); s, sin (Lat. *sinister*)
let a cerate be made ft cerat (Lat. *fiat ceratum*)
let a draught be made fh (Lat. *fiat haustus*)
let an emulsion be made ft emuls (Lat. *fiat emulsio*)
let an enema be injected inject enem (Lat. *injiciatur enema*)
let an enema be made ft enem (Lat. *fiat enema*)
let an eyewash be made ft collyr (Lat. *fiat collyrium*)
let a gargle be made ft garg (Lat. *fiat gargarisma*)
let him take it cap (Lat. *capiat*); su, sumat (Lat. *sumat*)
let an injection be made ft infus (Lat. *fiat infusum*)
let it be colored color (Lat. *coloretur*)
let it be continued pt (Lat. *perstetur*)
let it be digested dig (Lat. *digeretur*)
let it be dispensed disp (Lat. *dispensa, dispensetur*)
let it be dispensed quickly cit disp (Lat. *cito dispensatur*)
let it be divided d, div (Lat. *dividetur*)
let it be divided into equal parts d in p aeq (Lat. *dividetur in partes aequales*)
let it be done according to rule fla (Lat. *fiat lege artis*)
let it be given d, dent, det (Lat. *dentur, datur*); exhib (Lat. *exhibeatur*)
let it be given to dd (Lat. *datur ad*)
let it be given and labeled d et s (Lat. *datur et signetur*)
let it be given of such dose(s) dent tal dos (Lat. *dentur tales doses*)
let it be labeled sig (Lat. *signa, signetur*)

let it be made according to the rule fsar (Lat. *fiat secundum artem reglas*)

let it be made skillfully fsa (Lat. *fiat secundum artem*)

let it be reduced to powder redig in pulv (Lat. *redigatur in pulverem*)

let it be renewed ren (Lat. *renovetur*)

let it be repeated rep (Lat. *repetatur*)

let it be strained colet (Lat. *coletur*)

let it be swallowed deglut (Lat. *deglutiatur*)

let it be taken cap (Lat. *capiat*)

let it boil bull (Lat. *bulliat*)

let it not be repeated non rep, non repetat, nr (Lat. *non repetatur*)

let it to be taken as much as one wants to cap quant vult (Lat. *capiat quantum vult*)

let liniment be made ft linim (Lat. *fiat linimentum*)

let a mass be made ft mas (Lat. *fiat massa*)

let a mass be made and divided into pills ft mas div in pil (Lat. *fiat mass dividenda in pilulae*)

let medicine be continued cont rem (Lat. *continuetur remedium*)

let a mixture be made fm, ft mist (Lat. *fiat mistura*); m ft (Lat. *mistura fiat*)

let pills be made f pil (Lat. *fiat pilulae*)

let potion be made fp (Lat. *fiat potio*)

let a poultice be made ft cataplasm (Lat. *fiat cataplasma*)

let a powder be made ft pulv (Lat. *fiat pulvis*)

let it be reduced to powder redig in pulv (Lat. *redigatur in pulverem*)

let a solution be made ft solut (Lat. *fiat solutio*)

let a suppository be made ft suppos (Lat. *fiat suppositorium*)

let them stand st (Lat. *stent*)

let there be applied admov, admove (Lat. *admoveatur*)

let there be made ft (Lat. *fiat, fiant*)

let twice as much be given det in dup, det in 2 plo (Lat. *detur in duplo*)

light lev (Lat. *levis*)

liniment lin (Lat. *linimentum*)
liquid liq (Lat. *liquor*)
loose stools see *after very loose stools*
lotion lot (Lat. *lotio*)
lozenge troch (Lat. *trichiscus*)
lying down decub (Lat. *decubitus*)

M

macerate m, mac (Lat. *macerare*)
make see *let it be made, let there be made*
make a cerate see *let a cerate be made*
make an emulsion see *let an emulsion be made*
make an enema see *let an enema be made*
make an eyewash see *let an eyewash be made*
make a gargle see *let a gargle be made*
make an injection see *let an injection be made*
make pills see *let pills be made*
make a liniment see *let liniment be made*
make a mass see *let a mass be made*
make a mass and divide it into pills see *let a mass be made and divide it into pills*
make a mixture see *let a mixture be made*
make a poultice see *let a poultice be made*
make a powder see *let a powder be made*
make a solution see *let a solution be made*
make a suppository see *let a suppository be made*
make warm caf (Lat. *calefac*)
meal c (Lat. *cibus*)
   see also *after meals*
   see also *before meals and at bedtime*
   see also *between meals*
menses cta (Lat. *catamenia*)
mix m (Lat. *misce*)
mix and write label m et sig (Lat *misce et signa*)
mix very accurately m accur (Lat. *misce accuratissime*)
mix well mb (Lat. *misce bene*)
mix with caution m caute (Lat. *misce caute*)

mixture mist (Lat. *mistura*)
　see also *let a mixture be made*
morning man (Lat. *mane*)
　see also *at night and in the morning*
　see also *early in the morning*
　see also *every morning*
　see also *first thing in the morning*
　see also *in the morning*
　see also *morning and night*
　see also *to be taken tomorrow morning*
　see also *tomorrow morning*
morning and night m et n (Lat. *mane et nocte*)
mouth o (Lat. *os*)
　see also *by mouth*
　see also *nothing by mouth*
　see also *nothing by mouth at bedtime*
mouthwash collut (Lat. *collutorium*)
mustard sinap (Lat. *sinapis*)

N

nausea naus (Lat. *nausea*)
　see also *to the point of producing nausea*
near juxt (Lat. *juxta*)
neutralization see *to neutralization*
night noc (Lat. *nocte*)
　see also *at night*
　see also *at night and in the morning*
　see also *during the night*
　see also *every night*
　see also *every other night*
　see also *morning and night*
　see also *night and day*
　see also *six times a night*
　see also *three times a night*
　see also *to be taken tomorrow night*
　see also *tomorrow night*
night and day n et m (Lat. *nocte et mane*)

noon see *after noon*
  see *before noon*
note well nb (Lat. *nota bene*)
nothing by mouth npo (Lat. *nulla per os*)
nothing by mouth at bedtime npo/os (Lat. *nulla per os hora somni*)
number No, no (Lat. *numero*)
nutmeg nm (Lat. *nux moschata*)

O

odoriferous odorat (Lat. *odoratus*)
of proper consistency deb spis (Lat. *debita spissutudine*)
of the same ejusd (Lat. *ejusdem*)
of stone lapid (Lat. *lapideus*)
of whatever you please cuj lib (Lat. *cujus liber*)
of which cuj (Lat. *cujus*)
oil ol (Lat. *oleum*)
ointment ung (Lat. *unguentum*)
on alternate days dieb alt (Lat. *diebus alternis*)
once a day see *daily*
one hundred C (Lat. *centum*)
one half see *half*
orally see *by mouth*

P

pain dol (Lat. *dolor*)
  see also *to the painful side*
  see also *while pain lasts*
painful parts part dolent (Lat. *partes dolentes*)
paper chart (Lat. *charta*)
  see also *waxed paper*
part par (Lat. *pars*)
  see also *equal parts*
part affected par aff (Lat. *pars affecta*)
pill pil (Lat. *pilula*)

    see also *let a mass be made and divided into pills*
    see also *let pills be made*
pill mass mas pil (Lat. *massa pilularum*)
pint o (Lat. *octarius*)
plaster emp (Lat. *emplastrum*)
    see also *blistering plaster*
poison venen (Lat. *venenum*)
    see also *under poison label*
potion p (Lat. *potio*)
    see also *let potion be made*
poultice cataplasm (Lat. *cataplasma*)
    see also *let a poultice be made*
pour in inf (Lat. *infunde*)
pour off dec (Lat. *decanta*)
powder pulv (Lat. *pulvis*)
    see also *coarse powder*
    see also *let it be reduced to powder*
    see also *let a powder be made*
    see also *reduced to powder*
    see also *smooth powder*
    see also *very fine powder*
pregnancy grav (Lat. *gravitas*)
prescribe, prescription, prescription drug
    R_X (Lat. *recipe*)
    see also *last prescribed*
preserve see *keep*
proper consistency see *of proper consistency*
pure water aq pur (Lat. *aqua pura*)
purified dep (Lat. *depuratus*)

Q

quantity q (Lat. *quantum*)
quantity is correct qr (Lat. *quantum rectum*)
quantity not sufficient qns
    see also *sufficient quantity*
    see also *to sufficient quantity*
qualifications see *without other qualifications*

R

rectified spirit of wine svr (Lat. *spiritus vini rectificatus*)
rectally see *by way of rectum*
red rub (Lat. *ruber*)
reduce to powder see *let it be reduced to powder*
reduced to powder red in pulv (Lat. *reductus in pulverem*)
renew see *let it be renewed*
renew only once ren sem (Lat. *renovetum semel*)
repeat see *let it be repeated*
　　see *do not repeat*
right d, dex (Lat. *dexter*)
rub together conter (Lat. *contere*)

S

salt water bath bm (Lat. *balneum maris*)
same ead (Lat. *eadem*); id (Lat. *idem*)
　　see also *of the same*
sand bath BA (Lat. *balneum arenae*)
saturation see *to saturation*
scrapings rs (Lat. *rasurae*)
send mit (Lat. *mitte*)
send such doses mtd (Lat. *mitte tales doses*)
seven sept (Lat. *septem*)
shake agit (Lat. *agita*)
shake before taking agit ante sum (Lat. *agita ante sumendum*)
　　see also *first shake well*
six times a night sin (Lat. *sex in nocte*)
sleep see *every hour of sleep*
small cup pocill (Lat. *pocillum*)
so much of each ss (Gr. *ana*)
soap enema es (Lat. *enema saponis*)

smooth powder pulv subtil (Lat. *pulvis subtilis*)
soft moll (Lat. *mollis*)
soft capsule cap moll (Lat. *capsula mollis*)
solution sol (Lat. *solutio*)
  see also *let a solution be made*
spirit of vine sv (Lat. *spiritus vini*)
spoonful cochl (Lat. *cochleare*)
  see also *dessertspoonful*
  see also *heaping spoonful*
  see also *tablespoonful*
  see also *teaspoonful*
spray nebul (Lat. *nebula*)
sprinkle consperg (Lat. *consperge*)
steam bath bv (Lat. *balneum vaporis*)
stone see *of stone*
stools see *after very loose stools*
strain see *let it be strained*
strained colat (Lat. *colatus*)
strong fort (Lat. *fortis*)
such a one tal (Lat. *talis*)
sufficient quantity qs (Lat. *quantum satis*)
suppository suppos (Lat. *suppositorium*)
  see also *let a suppository be made*
swallow see *let it be swallowed*
syrup syr (Lat. *syrupus*)

T

tablet tab (Lat. *tabella*)
tablespoonful cochl mag (Lat. *cochleare magnum*)
take see *let him take it*
  see *let it be taken*
  see *to be taken*
taste see *to agreeable taste*
teaspoonful cochl inf (Lat. *cochleare infans*); cochl paarv
  (Lat. *cochleare parvum*)

tepid water aq tep (Lat. *aqua tepida*)

thickened by evaporation see *inspissated*

third day see *every third day*

this evening hoc vesp (Lat. *hoc vespere*)

three days trid (Lat. *triduum*)

three times a day, three times daily tid (Lat. *ter in die*); td (Lat. *ter die*)

three times a night tin (Lat. *ter in nocte*)

threshold l (Lat. *limen*)

throat gutt (Lat. *guttur*)

times vic (Lat. *vices*)

tincture tinc (Lat. *tinctura*)

to be added addend (Lat. *addendus*)

to agreeable acidity ad gr acid (Lat. *ad gratum aciditatem*)

to agreeable taste ad gr gust (Lat. *ad gratum gustum*)

to be administered adhib (Lat. *adhibentus*)

to be given dand (Lat. *dandus*)

to be taken capiend (Lat. *capiendus*); sum (Lat. *sumendus*)

to be taken as much as one wants to See *let it to be taken as much as one wants to*

to be taken four times a day qds (Lat. *quaque die sumendus*)

to be taken three times a day tds (Lat. *ter die sumendus*)

to be taken tomorrow morning cms (Lat. *cras sumendus*)

to be taken tomorrow night cns (Lat. *cras nocte sumendus*)

to be taken twice a day bds (Lat. *bis in die sumendus*)

to be used u, utend (Lat. *utendus*)

to fainting ad deliq (Lat. *ad deliquium*)

tomorrow see *for tomorrow*

see *to be taken tomorrow morning*

see *to be taken tomorrow night*

tomorrow morning cm (Lat. *cras mane*)

tomorrow night cn (Lat. *cras nocte*)

tonight hn (Lat. *hoc nocte*)

to neutralization ad neut (Lat. *ad neut*)

to the painful side lat dol (Lat. *lateri dolenti*); loc dol (Lat. *loco dolenti*)

to the point of fainting ad def an (Lat. *ad defectionem animi*)

to the point of producing nausea ad naus (Lat. *ad nauseum*)

to saturation ad sat (Lat. *ad saturandum*)

to sufficient quantity q sat (Lat. *quantum satis*)

to the throat gutt (Lat. *gutturi*)

to the weight of the whole ad pond om (Lat. *ad pondus omnium*)

toward the end of boiling sub fin coct (Lat. *sub finem coctionis*)

triturate trit (Lat. *tritura*)

trituration see *add trituration*

twice b, bis (Lat. *bis*)

twice a day bd (Lat. *bis die*); bid (Lat. *bis in die*)

twice a night bin (Lat. *bis in nocte*)

U

under poison label ssv (Lat. *sub signo veneni*)

until effective ad affect (Lat. *ad affectum*)

urethra see *by urethra*

use see *to be used*

V

vaginally see *by vagina*

vehicle see *in a suitable vehicle*

very fine powder pulv tenu (Lat. *pulvis tenuis*)

W

warmed calef (Lat. *calefactus*)
see also *make warm*

water A, AQ, aq (Lat. *aqua*)
  see also *add water*
  see also *cold water*
  see also *distilled water*
  see also *hot water*
  see also *in water*
  see also *pure water*
  see also *tepid water*
  see also *with water*
  see also *without water*
waxed paper chart cerat (Lat. *charta cerata*)
week hebdom (Lat. *hebdomas*)
weight see *by weight*
  see *to the weight of the whole*
well ben (Lat. *bene*)
when the action of emetic is over per op emet (Lat. *peracta operatione emetici*)
when bowels are constipated alv adst (Lat. *alva adstricta*)
when fever is coming on ag feb (Lat. *aggrediente febre*)
while fever is absent abs feb (Lat. *absente febre*)
while fever is present adst feb (Lat. *adstante febre*)
while fever lasts feb dur (Lat. *febre durante*)
while pain lasts dur dol (Lat. *durante dolor*)
white alb (Lat. *albus*)
with c (Lat. *cum*)
with a few drops gutt quibusd (Lat. *guttis quibvusdam*)
with proper direction dir prop (Lat. *directione propria*)
with the same amount ctant (Lat. *cum tanto*)
with water cum aq (Lat. *cum aqua*)
without sin (Lat. *sine*)
without expressing s expr (Lat. *sine expressio*)
without other qualifications sai (Lat. *sine altera indicatione*)
without water sin aq (Lat. *sine aqua*)

Y

yellow flav (Lat. *flavus*); lut (Lat. *luteus*)